What You Can Do for Her When She's Expecting

David Dunton

Illustrations by Harry Trumbore

RENAISSANCE BOOKS
Los Angeles

for Noah

Library of Congress Cataloging-in-Publication Data
Dunton, David.
     What you can do for her when she's expecting / David Dunton ; illustrations by Harry Trumbore.
          p. cm.
     ISBN 1-58063-055-3 (alk. paper)
     1. Pregnancy—Humor. 2. Pregnant women—Humor. 3. Husbands—Humor. I. Title.
PN6231.P68D86   1999
741.5'973—dc21   98-50125
                                                          CIP

10 9 8 7 6 5 4 3 2 1
Design by Lisa-Theresa Lenthall
Distributed by St. Martin's Press
Manufactured in the United States of America
First Edition

Acknowledgments

Thanks for advice and friendship on matters pre-parental and otherwise to Chris Harford, Debbie Chapman, Michael Hill, Grant Blaisdell, Dave Stern, Kate M. Ryan, Lillian Rosenblatt C.S.W., Liza Karsten A.C.S.W., Eddie Joskow, Susan Dunton, Ed and Suzy Dunton, John Dunton, Harvey Klinger, and various online penpals. Thanks also to Michael Levine and Joe McNeely at Renaissance Books for their faith in this concept, to Kimbria Hays for all her help, and to Arthur Morey and Lisa Lenthall for making it look right.

A tip of the hat to Harry Trumbore for providing such a lively, fun, and appropriate vision to one-third of the book's suggestions.

Many thanks to superagent (and superfriend) Laurie E. Liss for believing in this project and having the courage to take on a "client" whose office is ten feet from her own.

Finally, to the woman who got the ball rolling, so to speak—Regina, love of my life, mother of Noah. Thank you for allowing me to "experiment" on you with some of these ideas, for providing the list of what not to say or do for a pregnant woman, for editorial comments, and for being such an excellent partner. It goes without saying that this book never would have come about without you.

*I*ntroduction

This book started popping out of me around the time something similar was happening to my four-months-pregnant wife. As she was experiencing all sorts of changes to her body, hormonal level, and psyche, I very quickly discovered the cocktail of emotions that accompanies the knowledge that your wife or partner or friend is pregnant—joy, sheer terror, and most profoundly, absolute helplessness.

This is the beginning of a great adventure.

Am I a third wheel here or what?

Can I be remotely useful?

At first it seems that there is simply *nothing* you can do that will help this person along in her forty-week baby-making production. It's obvious she could use an encouraging word or two, but beyond that, what can you do that will make her feel better?

As we went along, I continually discovered—either on my own, or through suggestions from friends, relatives, complete strangers, and oftentimes my wife—little things that helped. That is, helped both of us. Things that made her feel better, and things that made me feel better about this imbalance of duties. *Honey, while you're creating this life form, I'll be over in the corner, twiddling my thumbs. Let me know if I can help.* I desperately wanted to play a part in the process which I helped create, feel important, be helpful, and above all, I wanted to ease her discomfort. The "activities" I write about here helped me achieve all these goals.

Common sense is helpful, but it will only take you part of the way. As with most things in life, if you're blessed with at least a few dollops of the stuff, you'll be able to take one look at her and realize, *Uh, she'd probably appreciate it if I made dinner and insisted on cleaning up afterward.* But while it's true that your instincts might come in handy, this book is less about those moments of simple Gump-like brilliance and more about the out-of-left-field stuff— those things you might not necessarily think of—ideas of the *Would-you-please-arrange-all-the-pens-by-height-and-sort-them-by-color?* variety.

At all times the best advice is simply to stay on your toes, and be open to (and good humored about) any requests. *What's that?*

You'd like me to clean the corners of the refrigerator shelves after I'm finished hand-combing the shag carpet? No problem!

There are undoubtedly many other things you can think to do for the pregnant person in your life. *What You Can Do for Her When She's Expecting* is just to get you started. Do not perform these tasks in the hope of getting a pat on the head; likewise, try not to get discouraged if she doesn't like one or any number of the things you've done. Whatever you do, don't try using this book as a checklist— you'll wind up too exhausted (and broke) to be even remotely patient and good-natured. Just be as selfless as possible and remember that the end reward is, by far, the best thing in the world. Soon enough, the pregnant person in your life will be The Person Formerly Known as Pregnant, and she'll have a little bundle of trainable joy in her arms. But that's another story.

Now, what to do.

*A*nything she asks. . .

Bring her saltines each morning.

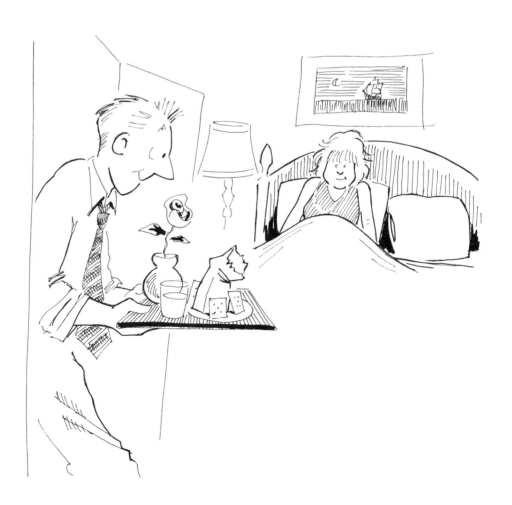

Don't complain about the crumbs in the bed.

Brush the crumbs out of the bed.

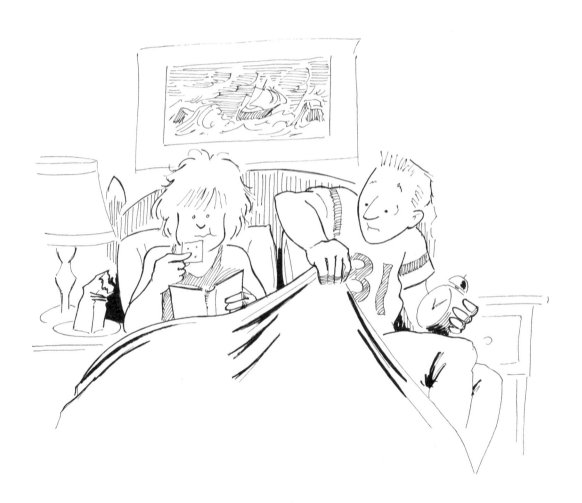

*A*ny time during the first trimester that your patience is tried, remember, SHE'S BUSY MAKING PLACENTA!

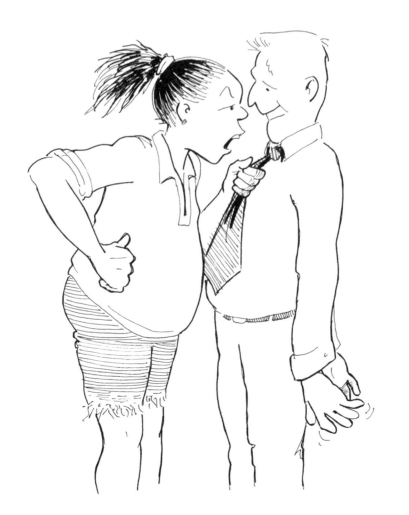

Draw a bath for her (not too warm)—add some bath salts, light a few candles, and then get out of her way so she can enjoy the experience.

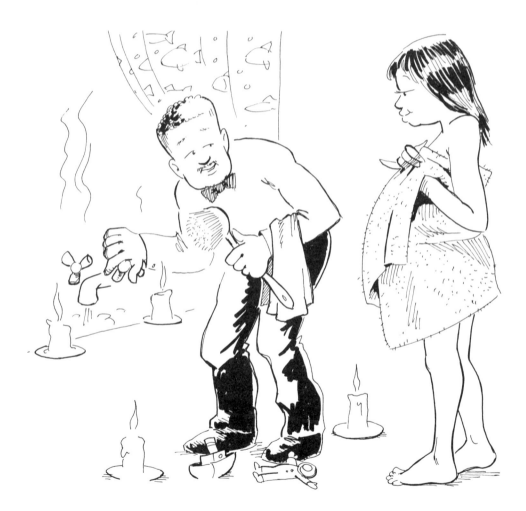

On your way out of the bathroom, take and then lose the scale.

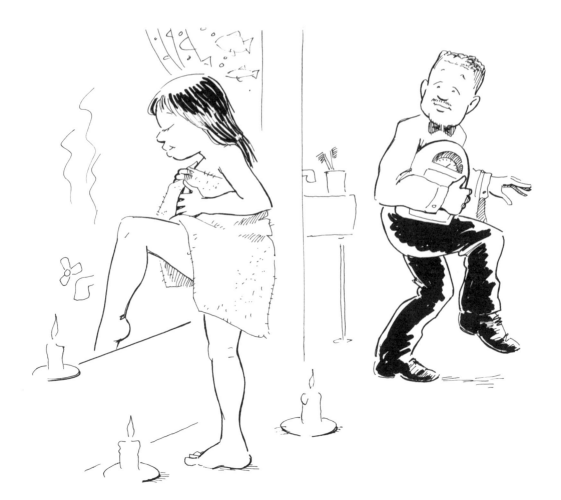

Baby her, but don't treat her like a baby.

• • •

Rub her back.

*T*ell her you love her. OFTEN.

Do not, under any circumstances, pressure her to have sex.

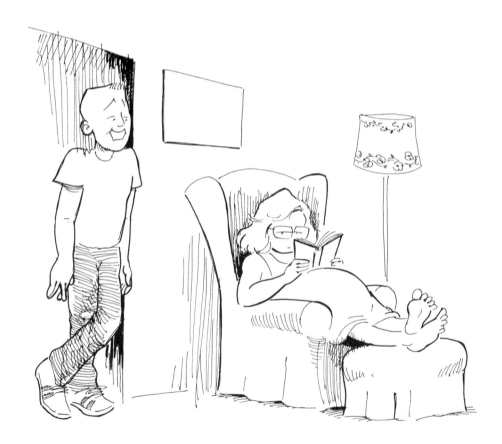

Flowers.

If she snaps at you, remind yourself that it's the hormones talking.

Buy her a body pillow. Encourage her to name it.

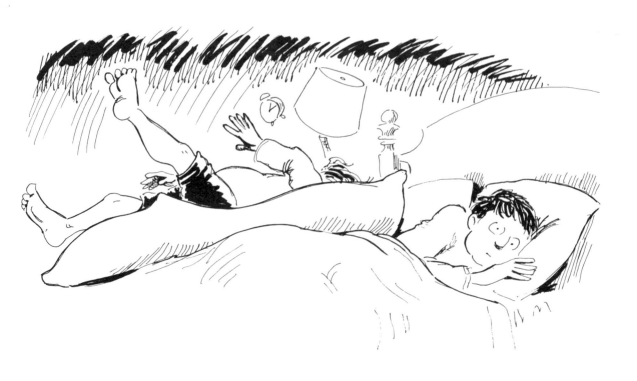

Gently run your fingers through her hair.

. . .

If she hollers, let it go.

. . .

*Let her hit you if she feels the urge.
Then go hide.*

Do as many of the household chores as you can handle. If there are things you don't know how to do, now's the time to learn.

If you're at all sick, STAY AWAY. This applies to any moment while she's pregnant.

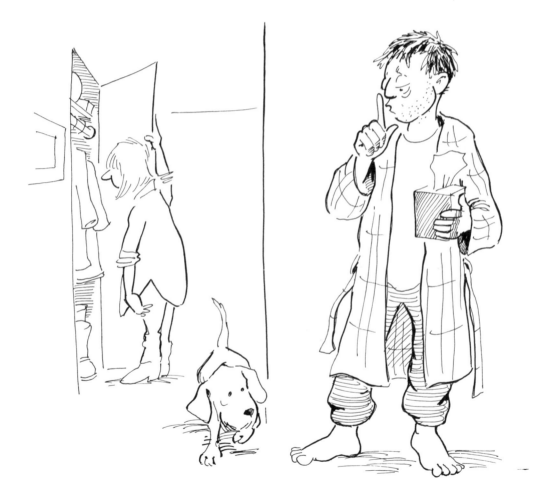

Give her a gift certificate for a hair appointment.

Give her a gift certificate for a manicure.

Give her a gift certificate for a pedicure.

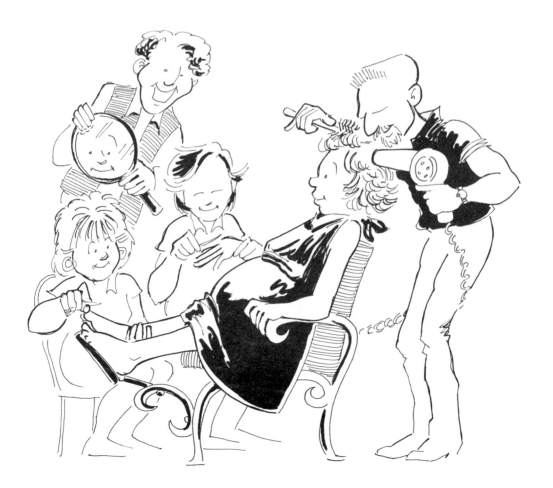

Stock the cabinets and refrigerator with at least one of everything for those spur-of-the-moment cravings.

•   •   •

Continue to encourage her to eat anything she wants. Chances are her body knows what it needs.

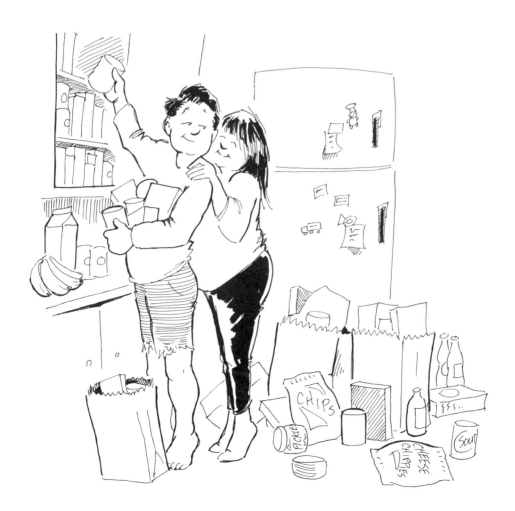

Become the model of versatility.

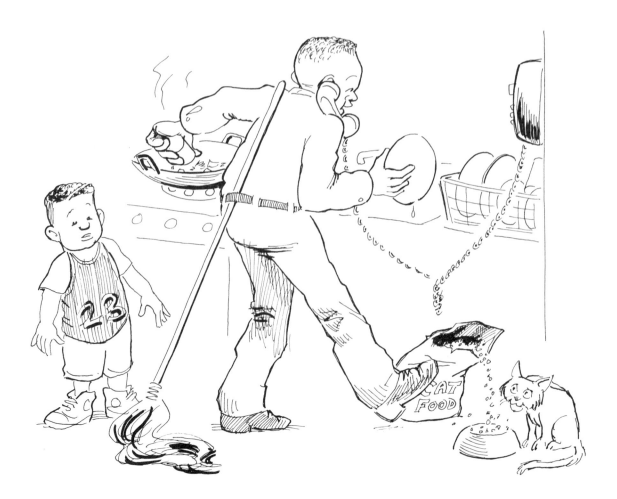

NEVER let her change the cat's litter box during the pregnancy.

(Seriously!)

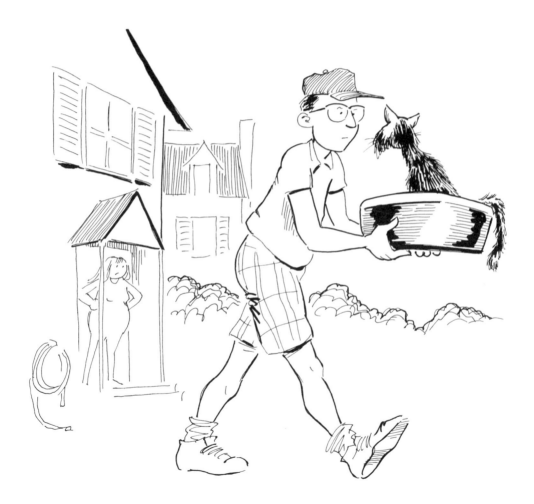

Keep plenty of ice water on hand.

And citrus foods.

*A*nd sweets.

*A*nd, of course, savories.

Gather as many take-out menus as possible.

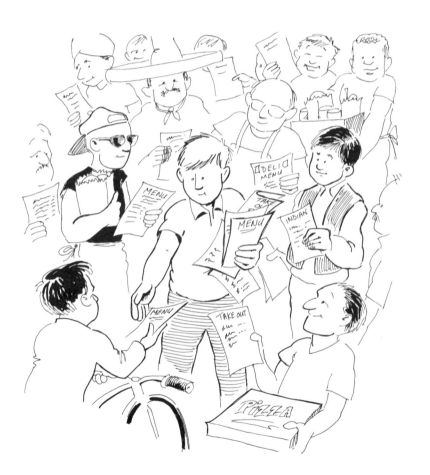

Invite her out for a walk; then let her set the pace.

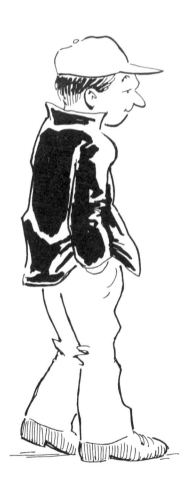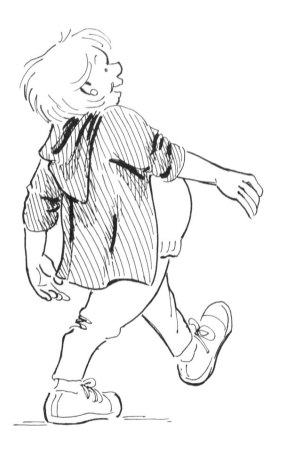

Don't ask; just hire someone to do the cleaning for the last month or two.

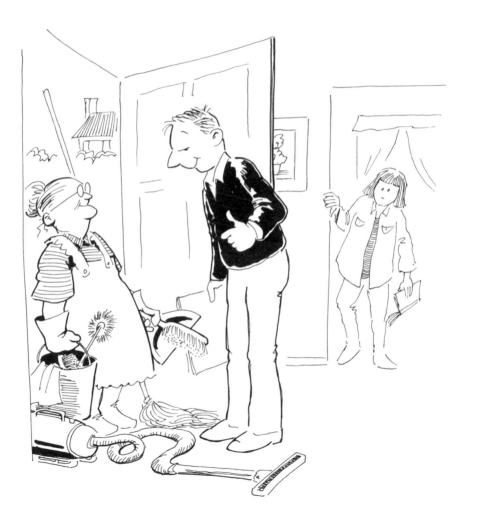

Do all household chores that require bending.

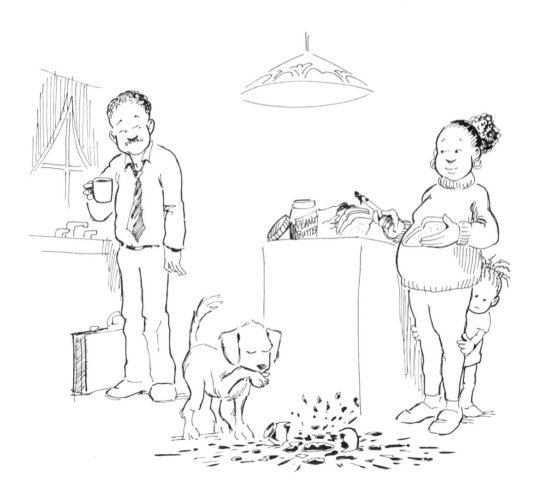

Never ever insist on doing, helping, holding, carrying, etc. If she wants something, she'll undoubtedly let you know.

•   •   •

Never try to convince her—in fact, don't even mention—that you wish you could be the one who was carrying the baby. You can't. You're not.

Give her a massage (or at least an appointment for one).

• • •

More flowers.

Peppermint foot oil, followed by a foot massage.

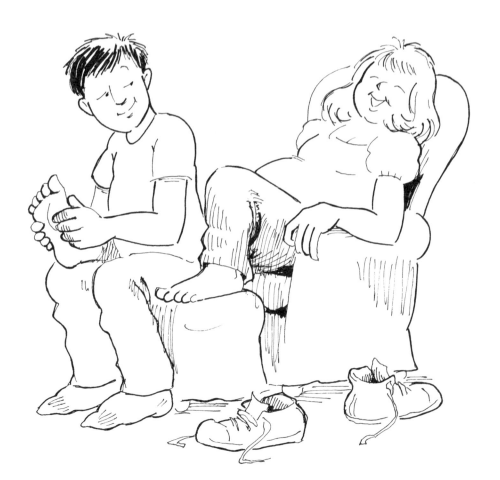

While you're getting used to the idea of the forthcoming kid, don't forget—she's already way ahead of you.

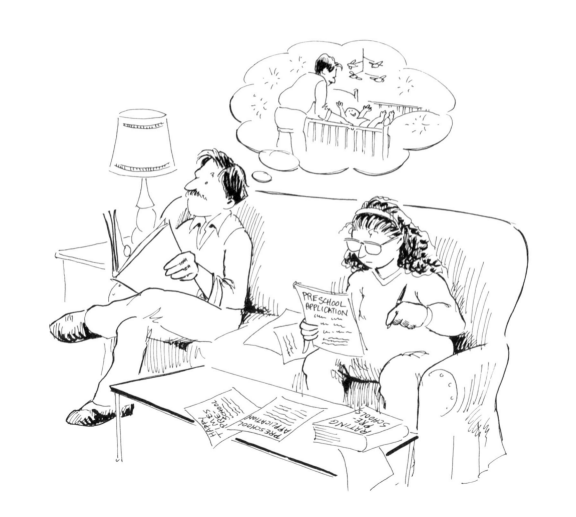

*Be prepared but don't act surprised
if she wants to have sex.*

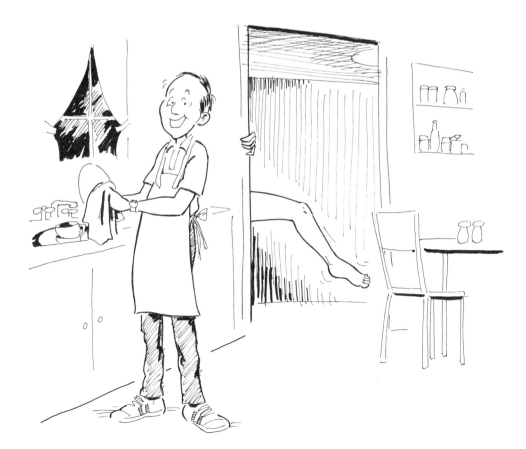

Tell her how sorry you are that she's feeling so sick.

• • •

More back rubs.

Ben & Jerry's™.

Buy her some body lotion that's "guaranteed" to ward off stretch marks. Put it on her if she allows.

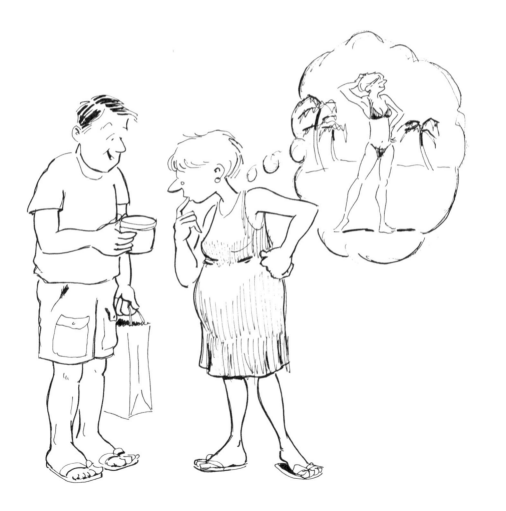

One, two, buckle or tie her shoe.

Three, four, open her door.

Five, six, take her to the flicks.

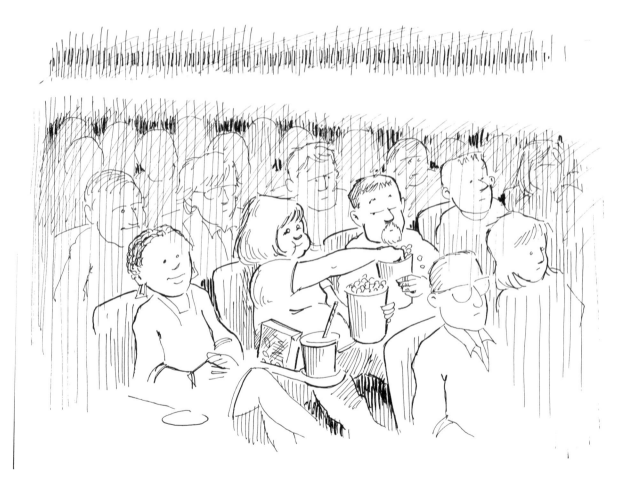

Seven, eight, don't ask about her weight.

Nine, ten, start this list again.

Go on vacation while you still have the time, inclination, and energy.

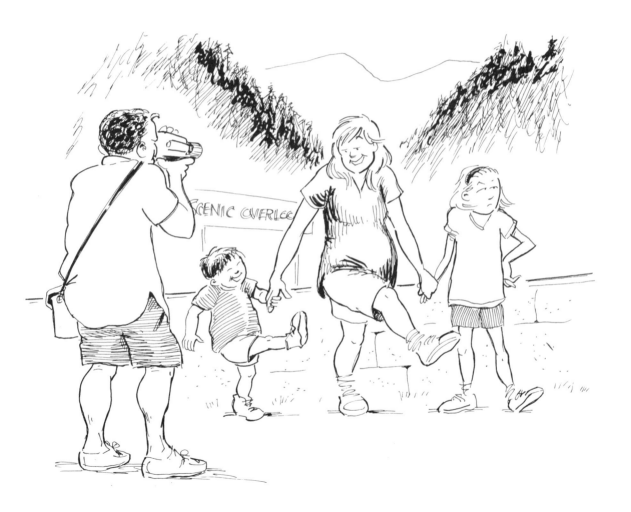

Tell her she looks great.

•   •   •

Listen when she needs to talk—don't try to "fix" what's wrong.

Even though you can't empathize, you can sympathize.

· · ·

Maintain an extra dose of patience at all times.

· · ·

Be understanding—even when you don't have a clue.

*A*sk to go with her to her doctor visits.
WANT TO GO.

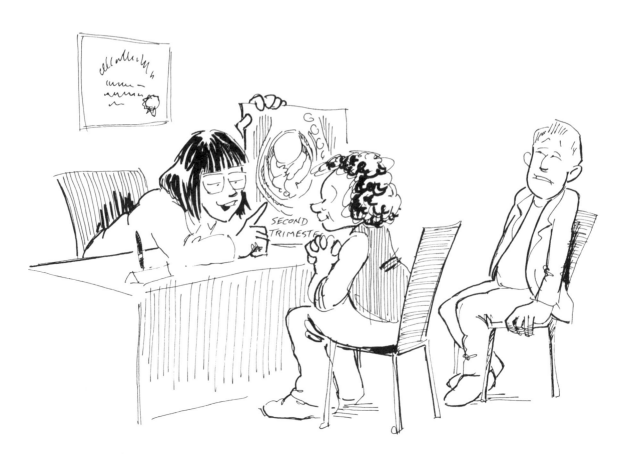

Since some women experience a touch of attention deficit disorder during pregnancy, bring her magazines (and not just pregnancy ones) and other things that can be read quickly.

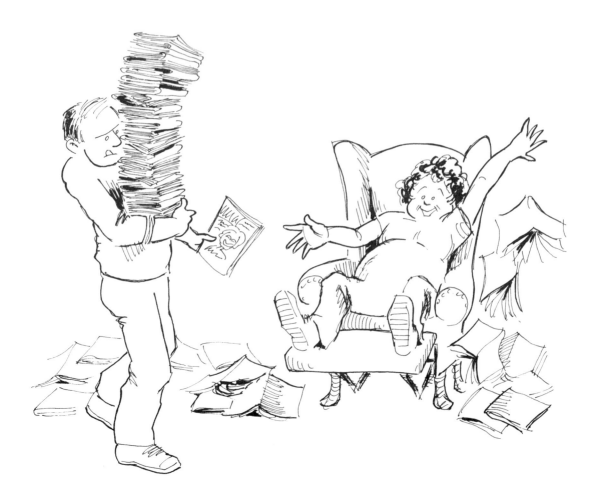

Encourage her to learn to squat—and to do it a lot. (This will help with the birth.)

Squat with her.

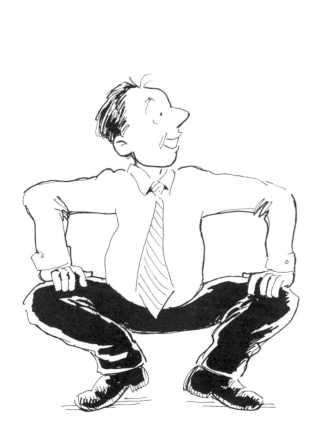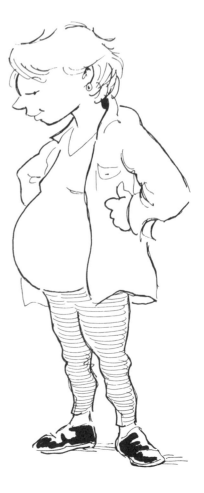

Her newly acute sense of smell might well have been crafted for the Bionic Woman. Be aware, and always carry a toothbrush and paste.

•   •   •

Don't take it personally if she uses the most efficient, if not polite, method of communication.

In the last month, stay within a half hour's distance from your hospital.

Always be reachable by phone, especially during the last month.

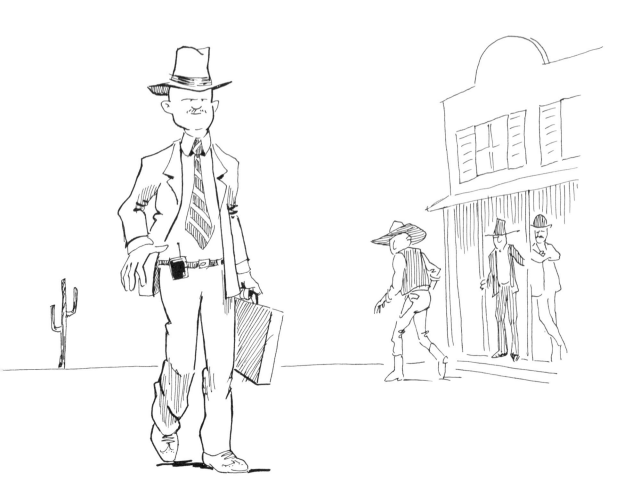

*F*ill a clean tube sock with uncooked rice and stitch it shut. Heat it in a microwave oven for three minutes—it will retain its heat for a long time. This makes for a great, flexible "heating pad" during labor (or any other time it's needed).

Get her a good, comfortable rocking chair.

Give her the gift of a maternal fitness or yoga class.

And when classes are done, gently remind her to do the exercises (as long as you feel certain she won't resort to physical violence when you do).

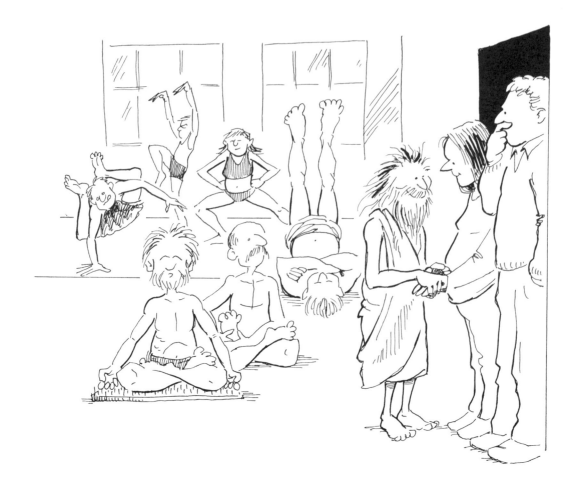

Give yourselves a childbirth and child-care class together. They take some of the edge off the uncertainty.

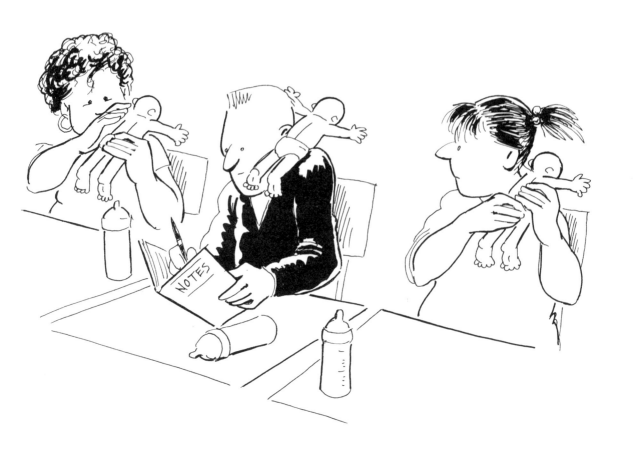

*T*ake her away for the weekend.

• • •

*L*eave her alone when she wants to be left alone, and don't take it personally.

• • •

*E*njoy your time alone together—while you still can.

Let her sleep!

Brush up on the rules for Yahtzee™, Scrabble™, all board games, gin rummy, and any other possible distractions.

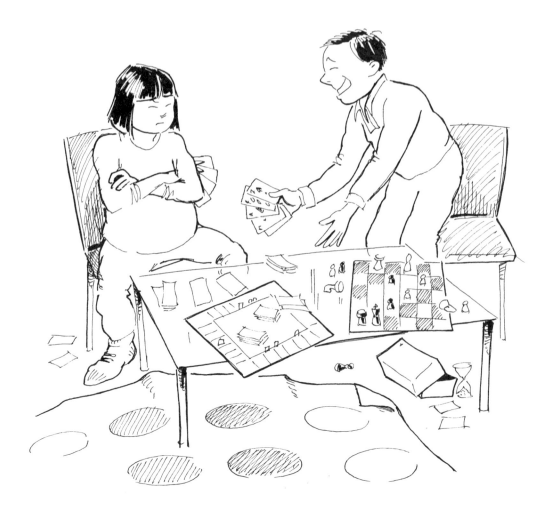

*D*on't make her necessary abstinence from coffee, cigarettes, alcohol, etc., more difficult by doing all three at the same time right in front of her.

• • •

*N*o matter that you think she's beautiful, SHE MAY NOT. Keep in mind what's happening to her body.
IT'S STILL HER BODY . . .

She is going to feel extremely fat and possibly ugly at times. Even though we may feel that pregnant women are really great, and quite beautiful, you are going to have to remember to constantly remind her of that. Got it?

Don't expect to be rewarded for good behavior.

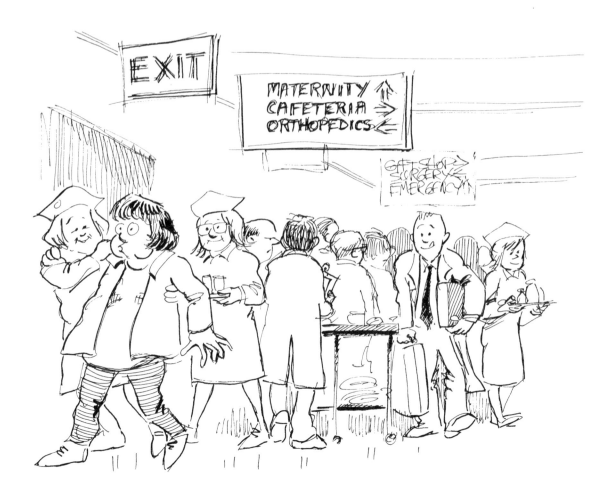

In the end, neither of you will remember any of these suggestions . . . until the next time.

Life will never be the same, but you're reading this, so believe me, it just gets better.

*T*he Ten Commandments of Keeping It Shut

Now that you know what to do, here are the ten commandments of what to absolutely not do. (These are only the choicest of the many stupid things that people—usually strangers—said to my wife when she was carrying our son.)

1. You are *huge!* Variation: I can't believe how big you're getting! That baby is going to be tremendous!

2. Haven't you had that baby yet? It seems like you've been pregnant forever!

3. Don't raise your arms above your head—the baby will strangle on its umbilical cord!

4. You know, you really shouldn't be eating/drinking that (fill in the blank).

5. Why are you still working? Shouldn't you be home resting?

6. Any horror story about someone else's pregnancy and/or labor (for example, stories about miscarriages, thirty-six-hour labors, etc.).

7. I'll bet you're having a girl, because you look really tired and girls steal your beauty.

8. It's too bad you're having a boy, because boys grow up and leave you.

9. You're so lucky that you're going to be on vacation (read: maternity leave) for three months!

10. What are you going to name your baby? Oh, that's very trendy right now.